I0704636

PSORIASIS FACTS

50 QUESTIONS ABOUT PSORIASIS ANSWERED!

(SIMPLIFIED)

By

Dr. Chris Allan

Copyright @ 2023 Dr. Chris Allan

All rights reserved.

Table of Contents

INTRODUCTION

One common misconception about psoriasis is that it is simply a cosmetic skin condition. However, psoriasis is a chronic autoimmune disorder that affects not only the skin, but also the joints and other parts of the body. Many people with psoriasis experience significant physical pain and discomfort, as well as emotional distress due to the visible symptoms of the condition.

Another misconception is that psoriasis is contagious and can be spread through physical contact. This is not true - psoriasis is not contagious and cannot be spread from person to person.

Many people also misunderstand the causes of psoriasis, believing it to be caused by poor hygiene or a lack of cleanliness. In reality, the exact cause of psoriasis is not known, but it is thought to be related to a combination of genetic and environmental factors.

Additionally, people often believe that psoriasis can be easily treated and cured, but this is not always the case. While there are a variety of treatments available, there is currently no cure for psoriasis, and treatment options can vary in their effectiveness for different individuals.

Psoriasis is often seen as something that only affects older people, while in reality, it can affect people of all ages, and it is not limited to certain racial or ethnic groups. In fact, psoriasis affects around 2-3% of the world population.

When Julie first noticed the red, flaky patches on her skin, she didn't think much of it. She assumed it was just a harmless rash and figured it would go away on its own. But as time went on, the patches grew larger and more numerous. Julie began to feel self-conscious and embarrassed about her appearance.

Feeling frustrated and desperate, Julie turned to the internet for answers. She scoured online forums and articles, trying to figure out what was wrong with her skin. She read about eczema, psoriasis, and a host of other skin conditions. But none of them seemed to match her symptoms exactly.

Eventually, Julie decided to visit a dermatologist. The doctor confirmed that she had psoriasis, a chronic autoimmune disorder that affects the skin. Julie was shocked and devastated. She had never heard of psoriasis before and had no idea how to deal with it.

Julie felt overwhelmed and alone. She isolated herself, avoiding social situations and hiding her skin under clothes and makeup. She even stopped going to work and school, convinced that people were staring at her and judging her.

But the more Julie avoided the outside world, the more her condition worsened. She became depressed and anxious, and her psoriasis only grew worse. Her self-esteem hit rock bottom and she felt like there was no way out.

Finally, Julie decided to seek help. She made an appointment with a therapist who specialized in helping people with psoriasis. The therapist helped Julie understand that psoriasis is not contagious and that people with psoriasis should not avoid social situations. She also recommended a support group for people with psoriasis, where Julie could connect with others who understood what she was going through. Through the group, Julie learned how to manage her symptoms, how to cope with the emotional toll of psoriasis, and how to maintain a positive outlook.

Over time, Julie began to feel better about herself. She stopped hiding and started to embrace her condition. She went back to work and school, and even started dating again. She realized that psoriasis did not define her as a person, it was just a part of her.

Many today may feel like Julie, depressed, frustrated and desperate because of this condition. But guess what! With the right knowledge, the right connections and community you find yourself you have little or nothing to worry. Its good you have taken out time to explore the facts about psoriasis and you'll be glad you did. This question and answer book for psoriasis covers all you need to know and in the course of my profession I have come to know and believe that the quickest way to learn is to ask questions and get the answers, these answers stay with you a life time.

SECTION 1

KNOW ABOUT PSORIASIS

1. What is Psoriasis?

Psoriasis is a chronic skin condition characterized by red, scaly patches on the skin. It is caused by an over-active immune system that causes the skin cells to grow too quickly. The patches, called plaques, can appear anywhere on the body, but are most commonly found on the scalp, knees, elbows, and lower back. Symptoms can include itching, burning, and soreness. While there is no cure for psoriasis, it can be managed with a variety of treatments including topical creams, light therapy, and oral medications. It is important to work with a dermatologist to develop an individualized treatment plan.

2. What are the symptoms of Psoriasis ?

The most common symptoms of psoriasis include:

Red, scaly patches on the skin: These patches are typically found on the scalp, elbows, knees, and lower back. They may be raised and thickened, and they may be covered with silvery scales.

Itching and burning: Many people with psoriasis experience itching and burning sensations on the affected areas of the skin.

Dry, cracked skin: Psoriasis can cause dry, cracked skin that may bleed or become infected.

Joint pain and stiffness: About 30% of people with psoriasis develop a form of arthritis called psoriatic arthritis, which causes pain and stiffness in the joints.

Nail changes: Psoriasis can cause changes in the nails, such as pitting, thickening, and discoloration.

Fatigue: Many people with psoriasis experience fatigue and a general feeling of being unwell.

In addition to these common symptoms, there are several different types of psoriasis, each with its own unique symptoms.

Plaque psoriasis: This is the most common form of psoriasis and is characterized by red, scaly patches on the skin.

Guttate psoriasis: This type of psoriasis is characterized by small, red, scaly spots on the skin. It often develops in childhood or young adulthood.

Inverse psoriasis: This type of psoriasis is characterized by red, smooth patches of skin in the folds of the body, such as the armpits, groin, and under the breasts.

Pustular psoriasis: This type of psoriasis is characterized by red, scaly patches on the skin that are filled with pus.

Erythrodermic psoriasis: This is a rare and severe form of psoriasis that covers most of the body with a red, peeling rash.

Psoriatic arthritis: This is a form of arthritis that occurs in people with psoriasis. It causes pain and stiffness in the joints and can lead to joint damage.

3. What are the different types of Psoriasis?

There are several different types of psoriasis, each with their own unique symptoms and characteristics.

Plaque Psoriasis: This is the most common type of psoriasis and is characterized by red, raised, and scaly patches on the skin. These patches, known as plaques, are typically found on the elbows, knees, scalp, and lower back, but can appear anywhere on the body. Plaque psoriasis can cause itching and pain, and in severe cases can lead to joint problems.

Guttate Psoriasis: This type of psoriasis is characterized by small, red, scaly patches that are typically found on the trunk and limbs. Guttate psoriasis is more common in children and young adults, and is often triggered by a bacterial infection such as strep throat.

Inverse Psoriasis: This type of psoriasis is characterized by red, shiny, and smooth patches of skin that are typically found in areas where the skin rubs together, such as the armpits, groin, and under the breasts. Inverse psoriasis can be painful and itchy, and is often made worse by sweating and friction.

Pustular Psoriasis: This type of psoriasis is characterized by red, raised, and scaly patches of skin that are filled with small, white, pus-filled blisters. Pustular psoriasis can be found on any part of the body, but is most common on the palms of the hands and the soles of the feet. This type of psoriasis can be very severe and can cause fever, chills, and overall feelings of sickness.

Erythrodermic Psoriasis: This is a rare and severe form of psoriasis characterized by a widespread redness and scaling of the skin. Erythrodermic psoriasis can cause fever, chills, and a fast heart rate, and can be life-threatening if not treated promptly.

Psoriatic Arthritis: This type of psoriasis is characterized by inflammation and pain in the joints, in addition to the skin symptoms of psoriasis. Psoriatic arthritis can cause stiffness, pain, and difficulty moving the affected joints. It can occur in any joint of the body, and in some cases, it can cause severe joint damage and disability.

Nail Psoriasis: This type of psoriasis affects the nails and is characterized by thickened, discolored, and sometimes misshapen nails. Nail psoriasis can also cause the nails to separate from the nail bed, and can be painful.

Scalp Psoriasis: This type of psoriasis affects the scalp and is characterized by red, scaly, and sometimes itchy patches on the scalp. Scalp psoriasis can also cause hair loss, and in severe cases, can cause the scalp to become covered in thick, white scales.

4. What causes Psoriasis?

The exact cause of psoriasis is not fully understood, but recent research has provided new insights into the underlying mechanisms of the condition.

One of the main causes of psoriasis is believed to be a *genetic predisposition.* Studies have shown that certain genes are more commonly found in individuals with psoriasis, indicating that the condition may be inherited. Additionally, family history is a risk factor for developing psoriasis, with people with a parent or sibling with psoriasis having a higher chance of developing the condition themselves.

The *immune system* also plays a crucial role in the development of psoriasis. Research has found that psoriasis is caused by a malfunction in the immune system, which leads to an overactive response in the skin. This overactive response causes skin cells to grow and divide at an accelerated rate, leading to the formation of plaques on the skin.

A key component of the immune response in psoriasis is the *activation of T cells*, a type of white blood cell. T cells normally help the body to fight off infections, but in psoriasis, they mistakenly attack healthy skin cells, leading to inflammation and the formation of plaques. This overactivation of T cells is believed to be caused by a dysfunction in the signaling pathways that regulate their activity, which is why this type of cells can develop in numbers that cause such issue.

Another aspect that is believed to contribute to psoriasis is a *dysfunction in the skin barrier*. The skin barrier is responsible for protecting the body from external stressors and maintaining hydration levels in the skin. In psoriasis, the skin barrier is damaged, allowing harmful bacteria and other irritants to penetrate the skin, which can lead to inflammation and further exacerbation of the condition.

Stress is also believed to be a key factor in the development and progression of psoriasis. Studies have shown that stress can trigger psoriasis flares and exacerbate the condition. Stress activates the sympathetic nervous system, which can lead to an increase in pro-inflammatory cytokines in the skin, exacerbating the immune response and causing the formation of plaques.

Environmental factors also play a role in the development of psoriasis. Exposure to environmental toxins such as pollutants and smoking can increase the risk of developing psoriasis. Additionally, certain medications such as lithium, beta blockers, and antimalarials can also trigger psoriasis or worsen existing symptoms.

In recent years, researchers have identified new pathways that contribute to psoriasis, including the role of the *gut microbiome*. Studies have found that individuals with psoriasis have a different composition of gut bacteria compared to individuals without the condition. This suggests that the gut microbiome may play a role in the development of psoriasis.

Moreover, new data found that there is a relationship between psoriasis and other chronic conditions such as obesity, metabolic syndrome, and cardiovascular disease. This suggests that psoriasis may be a manifestation of a *systemic inflammatory state,* rather than just a skin condition.

Finally, recent research has revealed new insights into the role of vitamin D in psoriasis. Vitamin D has been found to play a key role in regulating the immune response and is known to be a regulator of keratinocyte (skin cells) proliferation and differentiation. Studies have found that low levels of vitamin D are associated with an increased risk of psoriasis, and supplementing with vitamin D may help to reduce symptoms.

5. Is Psoriasis contagious?

Psoriasis is a skin condition that lasts for a long time and is not contagious. It is brought on by a combination of genetic and environmental factors. It cannot be spread from one person to another and is not brought on by poor hygiene or lifestyle choices.

Contact cannot spread the disease from one person to another. It cannot, like a cold or the flu, be "caught."

Instead, it is thought that psoriasis is brought on by a mix of genetic and environmental factors. Psoriasis is more common in those with a family history, and certain triggers, such as stress, infection, skin injury, and certain medications, can exacerbate the condition in those with it. The fact that psoriasis can affect the skin in a way that makes it look infected or dirty may be the source of the misconceptions about the condition. However, the symptoms are not brought on by an infection but rather by the rapid accumulation of skin cells.

Psoriasis affects more than just the skin; it can also affect the nails, scalp, and, in severe cases, the joints, resulting in Psoriatic Arthritis.

To help lessen the stigma associated with psoriasis, it is essential to educate oneself and dispel any erroneous notions about the condition.

6. Is there a link between Psoriasis and other health conditions?

Research has shown that people with psoriasis have an increased risk of developing other health conditions, including:

Cardiovascular disease: Studies have found that people with psoriasis have a higher risk of heart attack, stroke, and other cardiovascular problems. This may be due to the inflammation associated with psoriasis, as well as other risk factors such as obesity and smoking.

Metabolic syndrome: People with psoriasis are more likely to have metabolic syndrome, a group of conditions that includes high blood pressure, high blood sugar, and abnormal cholesterol levels. This can increase the risk of heart disease and diabetes.

Psoriatic arthritis: Up to 30% of people with psoriasis develop a form of arthritis called psoriatic arthritis. This condition causes inflammation and damage to the joints, leading to pain, stiffness, and decreased mobility.

Depression and anxiety: People with psoriasis may be more likely to experience mental health problems such as depression and anxiety, which can affect their quality of life. This may be due to the physical and emotional impact of living with a visible and chronic condition.

Other skin conditions: People with psoriasis may also be at risk of developing other skin conditions such as eczema, rosacea, and seborrheic dermatitis.

It's important to note that not every person with psoriasis will develop these conditions, and people without psoriasis may develop these conditions. However, people with psoriasis should be aware of these increased risks and take steps to reduce their risk of developing these conditions. This can include maintaining a healthy lifestyle, such as eating a balanced diet, exercising regularly, and not smoking.

If you have psoriasis, it's important to work with your healthcare provider to manage the condition, and to be aware of any signs or symptoms of other conditions that may develop. Regular checkups, including skin exams and screenings for other conditions, can help detect and treat any issues early on.

7. Can stress trigger a Psoriasis flare-up?

Stress can trigger a flare-up of psoriasis, a chronic skin condition characterized by red, scaly patches of skin. Studies have shown that stress can increase the production of inflammatory chemicals in the body, leading to an exacerbation of psoriasis symptoms.

There is a growing body of evidence linking stress to psoriasis flare-ups. Studies have shown that stress can increase the production of inflammatory chemicals, such as cytokines and tumor necrosis factor-alpha (TNF-alpha), which are known to play a role in the development of psoriasis. These chemicals contribute to the inflammation and abnormal skin cell growth associated with psoriasis.

In addition to its effects on inflammatory chemicals, stress can also affect the immune system, which is known to play a role in the development of psoriasis. Stress can lead to changes in the immune system, making it more susceptible to infections and inflammation. This can contribute to psoriasis flare-ups, particularly in people who have a genetic predisposition to the condition.

Moreover, stress can also affect mental health and increase the risk of depression and anxiety which in turn can exacerbate the symptoms of psoriasis. Studies have shown that people with psoriasis are more likely to experience mental health problems such as depression and anxiety and that these conditions can make psoriasis worse.

Stress can trigger a psoriasis flare-up. Studies have shown that stress can increase the production of inflammatory chemicals in the body and affect the immune system, leading to exacerbation of psoriasis symptoms. By managing stress through relaxation techniques, regular exercise, and a healthy diet, and seeking professional help for mental health conditions, individuals with psoriasis can reduce their risk of flare-ups and improve their overall health.

8. Can children get Psoriasis?

Yes, children can get psoriasis. Psoriasis is a chronic, inflammatory skin condition that affects approximately 2-3% of the population worldwide. It can affect people of all ages, including children. In fact, it is estimated that up to 10% of all psoriasis cases occur in children under the age of 10.

Symptoms of psoriasis in children can vary depending on the severity of the condition. Common symptoms include:

Red, scaly patches on the skin

Itching, burning, or stinging sensations

Thickened, cracked, or discolored nails

Painful, swollen joints (in cases of psoriatic arthritis)

Treatment options for children with psoriasis include:

Topical medications: These include creams, ointments, and gels that are applied directly to the skin. They can include corticosteroids, coal tar, and vitamin D analogues.

Phototherapy: This involves exposing the skin to specific types of ultraviolet light. UVB and PUVA are the most commonly used types of phototherapy for psoriasis in children.

Systemic medications: These medications are taken orally or by injection and are used to treat moderate to severe cases of psoriasis. They can include methotrexate, cyclosporine, and biologic drugs.

Lifestyle changes: Maintaining a healthy diet, avoiding smoking and alcohol, and practicing stress management techniques can help manage the symptoms of psoriasis in children.

It is important to note that children with psoriasis may experience emotional and social issues, as well. Children with psoriasis may feel self-conscious about their appearance and may be bullied or avoided by their peers. Parents should be aware of this and help their child feel positive about their skin.

9. Is there a genetic component to Psoriasis?

Yes, there is a significant genetic component to psoriasis. Studies have shown that individuals with a family history of psoriasis are more likely to develop the condition themselves. Additionally, specific genetic mutations have been identified as being associated with the development of psoriasis.

The most well-known genetic association with psoriasis is the presence of HLA-Cw6. This is a specific allele (variant) of the human leukocyte antigen (HLA) gene, which is involved in the immune system. Individuals who carry the HLA-Cw6 allele are at a significantly increased risk of developing psoriasis. In fact, this allele is found in up to 70% of individuals with psoriasis.

Another genetic association with psoriasis is the presence of certain variations in the IL-23 and IL-12 genes. These genes are involved in the regulation of the immune system, and have been found to be more common in individuals with psoriasis. Additionally, there are several other genes that have been associated with psoriasis, including IL-23R, CARD14, and ERAP1.

While there is a strong genetic component to psoriasis, it is important to note that genetics are not the only factor in the development of the condition. Environmental factors such as stress, infection, and certain medications can also trigger the onset of psoriasis.

In summary, the genetic component of psoriasis is well established, and there is a significant amount of research ongoing to further understand the specific genetic mutations and mechanisms associated with the development of the condition. This will help to improve the diagnosis and treatment options for those with psoriasis in future.

10. Can I wear make-up with Psoriasis?

Yes, you can wear makeup with psoriasis. However, it is important to take certain precautions to ensure that your makeup does not irritate your skin or worsen your symptoms.

First, it is important to make sure that your skin is well-moisturized before applying makeup. This will help to prevent dryness and flaking, which can make your psoriasis worse. It is also important to use makeup that is specifically formulated for sensitive skin, as these products are less likely to cause irritation.

Second, it is important to avoid using makeup that is heavy or thick, as this can clog your pores and exacerbate your psoriasis symptoms. Opt for lightweight, water-based makeup products that will not clog your pores.

Third, it is important to avoid using makeup products that contain fragrances or other harsh chemicals, as these can cause irritation and worsen your psoriasis symptoms. Look for makeup products that are fragrance-free and hypoallergenic.

Finally, it is important to remove your makeup gently and thoroughly at the end of the day. Use a gentle, non-irritating makeup remover and avoid scrubbing your skin too hard.

11. What food should a Psoriasis patient avoid?

While there is no specific diet that can cure psoriasis, certain foods may trigger or worsen symptoms in some individuals.

Some research suggests that a diet high in processed foods, sugar, and saturated fats may be associated with an increased risk of psoriasis. Therefore, it may be beneficial for those with psoriasis to limit their intake of these foods.

Additionally, some studies have found that a diet high in gluten, a protein found in wheat, barley, and rye, may be associated with a higher risk of psoriasis. Therefore, some people with psoriasis may benefit from a gluten-free diet. However, it's important to note that a gluten-free diet should only be followed under the guidance of a healthcare professional, as it can be low in important nutrients.

There are also some foods that have anti-inflammatory properties, which may help to reduce symptoms of psoriasis. These include fatty fish such as salmon and mackerel, which are high in omega-3 fatty acids, as well as fruits and vegetables, nuts, and seeds. It is also recommended to eat more of whole food which are less processed, non-GMO and organic as much as possible

In addition to avoiding certain foods, it's also important to maintain a healthy and balanced diet overall. This can include eating a variety of fruits, vegetables, whole grains, lean proteins, and healthy fats.

It is also important to note that, Everyone's symptoms and triggers for psoriasis are different so it is always a good idea to consult with a healthcare professional or a registered dietitian before making any major changes to your diet. They can help you create a meal plan that's tailored to your individual needs and can also help you monitor any changes in your symptoms.

It's also important to remember that diet alone may not be able to fully control psoriasis symptoms, and it's important to continue following any treatment plan prescribed by your healthcare provider.

12. Can I get a tattoo even with Psoriasis?

Yes, you can get a tattoo even if you have psoriasis. However, it is important to be aware of some considerations before getting a tattoo.

Firstly, it is important to note that psoriasis is a chronic condition that causes the skin to become red and scaly. The condition can also cause itching and pain, which can make getting a tattoo more uncomfortable. It is recommended that people with psoriasis speak with their doctor before getting a tattoo to ensure that the condition is well managed and that there are no open sores or flares on the area where the tattoo will be applied.

Secondly, it is important to choose a reputable tattoo artist who is aware of the risks associated with tattooing someone with psoriasis. They should be able to use appropriate precautions, such as using new needles, gloves and disposable razors, to prevent any further infection or worsening of the psoriasis. The tattoo artist should also be willing to work with you to minimize any discomfort or pain associated with the tattooing process.

Thirdly, it is important to be aware that getting a tattoo can cause psoriasis to flare up. This is because the tattooing process causes injury to the skin, which can trigger the immune system to respond and create new skin cells. This can cause a flare-up of psoriasis symptoms, such as redness and scaling, in the area where the tattoo was applied.

Some studies have shown that people with psoriasis are more likely to develop an infection after getting a tattoo, and are also more likely to experience issues with tattoo healing. This is because the condition can affect the skin's ability to heal properly.

13. Can I swim with Psoriasis?

Yes, you can swim with psoriasis. However, there are certain precautions that should be taken to prevent the condition from worsening.

Psoriasis is a chronic skin condition characterized by red, scaly, and itchy patches of skin. Swimming in a chlorinated pool can cause skin irritation and dryness, which can aggravate psoriasis symptoms. To prevent this, it is recommended to shower immediately after swimming to remove any chlorine residue on the skin. Applying a moisturizer or a mild lotion can also help to hydrate the skin and reduce itching.

Swimming in saltwater, on the other hand, can be beneficial for people with psoriasis. Saltwater is known to have anti-inflammatory properties and can help to reduce the redness and itching associated with psoriasis. Swimming in the ocean or a saltwater pool can also help to remove scales and flakes from the skin.

Another important consideration when swimming with psoriasis is sun exposure. Sunlight can aggravate psoriasis symptoms and increase the risk of skin cancer. It is recommended to use a sunscreen with an SPF of at least 30 to protect the skin while swimming. A sunscreen specifically formulated for sensitive skin or with physical blocks like zinc oxide is best for people with psoriasis. Swimming can be a beneficial form of exercise for people with psoriasis, but it is important to take precautions to prevent the condition from worsening. Showering immediately after swimming and using a moisturizer or lotion can help to hydrate the skin and reduce itching. Swimming in saltwater can also be beneficial for people with psoriasis, but it is important to use a sunscreen to protect the skin from sun exposure. It is always recommended to consult with your dermatologist before making any significant changes to your skincare routine.

14. How do I talk to my employer about my Psoriasis?

It can be difficult to talk to your employer about your psoriasis, but it is important to have an open and honest conversation about your condition and its impact on your work. Here are some practical tips for having this conversation:

Be prepared: Before speaking to your employer, it is important to have a clear understanding of your condition and how it affects you. This may include researching your condition, talking to your doctor, and identifying any accommodations or adjustments you may need in the workplace.

Schedule a meeting: Set up a meeting with your employer to discuss your condition and its impact on your work. Make sure to choose a time and location that is convenient for both of you.

Communicate clearly: Explain your condition and how it affects you, including any symptoms or triggers that may impact your work. Be sure to also mention any accommodations or adjustments you may need to help you manage your condition.

Be open to feedback: Your employer may have concerns or questions about your condition and its impact on your work. Be open to discussing these concerns and finding solutions together.

Provide documentation: It may be helpful to provide your employer with written documentation from your doctor, such as a note or letter detailing your condition and any accommodations or adjustments you may need.

Follow-up: After the meeting, follow up with your employer to ensure that any accommodations or adjustments have been put in place and to address any concerns or issues that may arise.

It's also worth mentioning that you have the right to reasonable accommodation under the Americans with Disabilities Act (ADA) and can request specific changes to help you perform your job more comfortably.

It's important to remember that your employer is required to provide reasonable accommodations to help you perform your job, so don't be afraid to ask for what you need. With open communication and a willingness to work together, you and your employer can find solutions to help you manage your psoriasis in the workplace.

15. What effect does exercise have on Psoriasis?

Exercise has been shown to have a positive effect on individuals with psoriasis. Regular physical activity can help to reduce symptoms, improve overall health, and boost self-esteem.

Firstly, exercise can help to reduce symptoms of psoriasis by decreasing inflammation throughout the body. Psoriasis is an autoimmune disorder characterized by inflammation and the overproduction of skin cells. Regular physical activity can help to reduce inflammation, which can lead to a reduction in symptoms such as redness, itching, and scaling.

Additionally, exercise can help to improve overall health. Physical activity can help to increase cardiovascular fitness, improve muscle strength, and promote weight loss. These health benefits can help to reduce the risk of other chronic health conditions such as obesity, diabetes, and heart disease.

Furthermore, exercise can also have a positive effect on mental health. Regular physical activity can help to reduce stress and anxiety, and improve overall well-being. This can be particularly beneficial for individuals with psoriasis, as stress and anxiety can trigger flare-ups.

Lastly, exercise can help to boost self-esteem and confidence in individuals with psoriasis. Physical activity can help to improve body image and self-perception, which can be particularly beneficial for individuals with visible skin conditions.

Therefore, exercise is a beneficial tool for individuals with psoriasis. Regular physical activity can help to reduce symptoms, improve overall health, and boost self-esteem. It is important to consult with a healthcare professional before starting an exercise routine, particularly if an individual has any underlying health conditions. Additionally, it is important to use sunscreen when engaging in outdoor activities, as exposure to UV radiation can worsen psoriasis symptoms.

16. Can I have a healthy pregnancy with Psoriasis?

Yes, it is possible to have a healthy pregnancy with psoriasis. However, it is important to work closely with your healthcare provider to manage your condition throughout your pregnancy.

Psoriasis is a chronic autoimmune disease that causes red, scaly patches on the skin. It can also cause joint pain and stiffness. Pregnancy can affect the severity of psoriasis, as hormonal changes can cause flare-ups or improvements in symptoms. Some women may experience worsening of their psoriasis during pregnancy, while others may have improvement.

It is important to note that certain medications used to treat psoriasis may not be safe to use during pregnancy. It is important to talk with your healthcare provider about alternative treatment options. For example, light therapy and topical creams may be safer options.

It is also important to maintain a healthy diet and exercise routine throughout your pregnancy. Eating a balanced diet and getting regular exercise can help to manage your psoriasis symptoms and improve overall health.

It is also important to address any emotional stress you may be experiencing during your pregnancy. Stress can exacerbate psoriasis symptoms, so it is important to find healthy ways to manage stress such as yoga, meditation, or therapy.

In general, most women with psoriasis can have healthy pregnancies, but it is important to work closely with your healthcare provider to manage your condition throughout your pregnancy. With the right treatment and support, you can successfully manage your psoriasis during pregnancy and have a healthy baby.

It is also important to be aware of any potential risks to your baby, such as pre-term birth or low birth weight, that may be associated with psoriasis. Your healthcare provider will be able to monitor your pregnancy and address any concerns you may have.

In summary, while psoriasis can be challenging to manage during pregnancy, it is possible to have a healthy pregnancy with the right treatment, support and close monitoring by healthcare providers. It is important to discuss any concerns you may have with your healthcare provider and to make sure you are following a healthy diet, exercise routine and managing stress. Your healthcare provider can help you to identify safe and effective treatment options, and to address any risks to your baby during pregnancy and delivery.

17. Does weather affect Psoriasis?

One question that is often asked by those who have psoriasis is whether weather can affect their condition.

The short answer is yes, weather can have an impact on psoriasis symptoms.

Cold and dry weather can be particularly problematic for those with psoriasis. When the air is dry, it can strip the skin of its natural moisture, which can lead to dry, cracked skin. This can make psoriasis symptoms worse, as dry skin is more likely to become irritated and inflamed. Cold weather can also cause the blood vessels in the skin to constrict, which can make the skin feel tighter and more itchy.

On the other hand, hot and humid weather can also be a problem for those with psoriasis. When the skin becomes overheated and sweat collects on the skin, it can lead to increased itching and irritation. This can be particularly problematic for those with severe psoriasis, as the increased inflammation can lead to the development of new plaques or the worsening of existing ones.

Sunlight can also have an impact on psoriasis symptoms. While moderate sun exposure can help to improve the condition of the skin, excessive sun exposure can lead to sunburn and damage to the skin. This can make psoriasis symptoms worse, as sunburned skin is more susceptible to inflammation and irritation.

So, what can be done to manage psoriasis symptoms during different weather conditions?

One of the most important things to remember is to keep the skin moisturized. This can be done by applying a thick, fragrance-free moisturizer to the skin at least twice a day. It's also important to avoid taking hot showers or baths, as they can strip the skin of its natural oils. Instead, take lukewarm showers or baths and limit the time spent in the water.

In hot and humid weather, it's important to keep the skin cool and dry. This can be done by wearing loose-fitting, breathable clothing and by staying out of the sun during the hottest parts of the day. It can also be helpful to use a fan or air conditioning to keep the air in the home cool and dry.

In cold and dry weather, it's important to keep the skin warm and moist. This can be done by wearing warm clothing and by using a humidifier in the home. It's also important to avoid long, hot showers or baths, as they can dry out the skin.

So, it's important to remember that everyone's skin is different and what works for one person may not work for another. It may take some trial and error to find the best ways to manage psoriasis symptoms during different weather conditions. It's also important to work with a dermatologist to find the best treatment plan for your individual needs.

18. Can I breastfeed with Psoriasis?

Yes, you can breastfeed with psoriasis. Psoriasis is a chronic skin condition that causes inflammation and redness on the skin. It is not contagious and does not affect the milk supply or quality of breast milk.

However, breastfeeding mothers with psoriasis may experience flare-ups in areas where the skin is stretched or chafed, such as the nipples or under the breast. It is important to keep these areas moisturized and protected to prevent cracking and soreness.

If you are experiencing a severe flare-up of psoriasis, it may be best to avoid breastfeeding until the condition improves. If you are taking medication for psoriasis, it is important to talk to your doctor about the potential risks of passing medication through breast milk to your baby.

It is also important to note that breastfeeding may help to improve your psoriasis symptoms by reducing stress and promoting relaxation. Studies have shown that breastfeeding may reduce the risk of developing psoriasis in the first place.

Overall, breastfeeding with psoriasis is possible, but it may require extra care to prevent flare-ups and soreness. It is important to talk to your doctor and a lactation consultant for personalized advice and support.

19. Can I drink alcohol with Psoriasis?

It is possible for individuals with psoriasis to drink alcohol, but it is important to be mindful of how it may affect the condition. Alcohol can exacerbate psoriasis symptoms, causing flare-ups and making it harder to manage the condition.

The relationship between alcohol and psoriasis is complex and varies from person to person. Research has shown that alcohol consumption can lead to an increased risk of psoriasis and a more severe form of the condition. This is believed to be due to the fact that alcohol can disrupt the balance of the immune system, which is already over-active in individuals with psoriasis.

Alcohol can also dehydrate the skin, making it more susceptible to dryness and itching, which are common symptoms of psoriasis. Additionally, alcohol can interfere with the effectiveness of medications used to treat psoriasis, such as methotrexate and acitretin.

It is important to note that different types of alcohol can have different effects on psoriasis. For example, beer and wine contain gluten, which can worsen symptoms for individuals with gluten sensitivities. Hard alcohol, such as whiskey and vodka, may be less likely to cause flare-ups, but it is still important to be mindful of how much is consumed.

Ultimately, the best approach is to monitor your symptoms closely and listen to your body. If you notice that drinking alcohol causes a flare-up of your psoriasis, it may be best to limit or avoid alcohol altogether. It is also important to speak with your doctor about how alcohol consumption may impact your treatment plan.

In summary, while it is possible for individuals with psoriasis to drink alcohol, it is important to be mindful of how it may affect the condition and speak with a doctor about potential impacts on treatment. Individuals with psoriasis should monitor their symptoms closely and make adjustments to their alcohol consumption as needed.

20. Can I smoke with Psoriasis?

Smoking with psoriasis can worsen the condition and potentially lead to further health complications.

Smoking is a known risk factor for psoriasis, as it can cause a flare-up of symptoms. This is because smoking causes inflammation in the body, which can worsen the inflammation associated with psoriasis. Additionally, smoking can also make psoriasis more difficult to treat. Studies have shown that smokers with psoriasis have a higher likelihood of developing more severe forms of the condition, such as psoriatic arthritis.

Smoking can also increase the risk of complications associated with psoriasis. For example, smokers with psoriasis are more likely to develop skin infections, and smoking can also increase the risk of cardiovascular disease, which is already higher in people with psoriasis.

It is important to note that smoking cessation is not a guaranteed cure for psoriasis, but it can significantly improve symptoms and reduce the risk of complications associated with the condition. Quitting smoking can also have numerous other benefits for overall health, including reducing the risk of lung cancer, heart disease, and stroke.

If you have psoriasis and smoke, quitting smoking should be a top priority. Your healthcare provider can help you find resources and support to quit smoking, such as nicotine replacement therapy and counseling. Additionally, they may also recommend other treatment options, such as topical creams, phototherapy, and medications, to help manage your psoriasis symptoms.

In conclusion, smoking can worsen psoriasis symptoms and increase the risk of complications associated with the condition. Quitting smoking is important for improving psoriasis symptoms and overall health. If you have psoriasis and smoke, speak with your healthcare provider to find resources and support to help you quit smoking and manage your psoriasis symptoms.

21. Can I use public pools with Psoriasis?

Yes, you can use public pools with psoriasis. However, it is important to take certain precautions to avoid exacerbating your condition.

First, it is important to avoid using any harsh chemicals, such as chlorine, that can irritate your skin. Instead, opt for pools that use salt water or mineral water. These types of pools are gentler on the skin and can even help to soothe symptoms of psoriasis.

Next, be sure to protect your skin from the sun. Psoriasis is a condition that can cause your skin to become more sensitive to UV rays. Apply sunscreen before entering the pool and wear protective clothing such as a rash guard or swim shirt to cover exposed skin.

It is also important to avoid scratching or rubbing your skin while in the pool. Psoriasis can cause itching, but scratching or rubbing can make the condition worse. Try to keep your skin moisturized before and after swimming to help alleviate itching and dryness.

Finally, be aware that public pools can be crowded and the water may not be as clean as you would like. Consider bringing your own towel and bathrobe to avoid coming into contact with bacteria or other contaminants that may be present in the water.

Ultimately, using public pools with psoriasis is possible as long as you take the necessary precautions to protect your skin. Seek advice from your dermatologist before swimming in any public pools or ocean. They will be able to recommend the best course of action for your individual case and help you manage your psoriasis more effectively.

22. How do I explain Psoriasis to my friends and family?

The first step in explaining psoriasis to your friends and family is to educate them about the condition. Provide them with information about what causes psoriasis, how it is diagnosed, and the different types of treatment available. Explain that psoriasis is not contagious, and that it is not caused by poor hygiene or lifestyle choices.

Next, it is important to address any misconceptions or stereotypes that your friends and family may have about psoriasis. For example, some people may believe that psoriasis is a minor skin condition, when in fact it can have a significant impact on a person's quality of life.

Others may think that psoriasis is contagious, when in fact it is not.

Another important step is to be open and honest about your own experiences with psoriasis. Share with your friends and family how the condition affects you, and how you manage it. This will help them to understand the challenges that you face, and to be more supportive of you.

It's also important to set realistic expectations with your friends and family. Explain that while there are effective treatments available, psoriasis is a chronic condition that cannot be cured. It may also be helpful to let them know that psoriasis symptoms may come and go and may not respond to treatment all the time.

As a matter of fact, it is essential to remind your friends and family that you are still the same person, regardless of your condition. Psoriasis is a part of who you are, but it does not define you. Encourage them to treat you with kindness and understanding, and to be supportive of you as you manage your condition.

So, educating your friends and family about psoriasis, addressing any misconceptions they may have, being open and honest about your own experiences, setting realistic expectations and reminding them that you are still the same person regardless of your condition are practical steps that can help you avoid stigmatization. With their support, you can manage your condition and live a fulfilling life.

23. How do I support a loved one with Psoriasis?

Educate yourself about psoriasis: Understanding the condition and its symptoms can help you empathize with your loved one and offer them the support they need. Read up on the different types of psoriasis, triggers, and treatment options.

Be patient and understanding: Psoriasis can be a frustrating and embarrassing condition for many people. Be patient with your loved one when they are feeling down or self-conscious about their appearance.

Help with practical tasks: Offer to help your loved one with tasks that may be difficult for them due to their psoriasis. This could include things like grocery shopping, cooking, or cleaning.

Encourage them to seek treatment: Help your loved one find a dermatologist or other healthcare professional who can provide them with appropriate treatment for their psoriasis. Encourage them to stick with their treatment plan and to speak with their doctor about any concerns they may have.

Be a listening ear: Psoriasis can be an emotional condition. Be there to listen to your loved one when they need to talk about their feelings or frustrations.

Be supportive of their self-care routine: Help your loved one develop a self-care routine that is tailored to their psoriasis. This may include things like regular moisturising, using sun protection, and avoiding triggers.

Help them find support groups: Many people with psoriasis find it helpful to connect with others who understand their condition. Help your loved one find local support groups or online communities where they can connect with others who have psoriasis.

Celebrate their successes: Encourage your loved one to celebrate their successes, no matter how small. This could be something as simple as having a good day with minimal symptoms or trying a new treatment that is working well.

Be sensitive to their feelings: Remember that psoriasis can be an emotionally taxing condition. Be sensitive to your loved one's feelings, and try not to say things that may make them feel self-conscious or ashamed.

Show them you love them: Above all, remember to show your loved one that you love and support them. Whether it's a simple hug or a heartfelt conversation, let them know that you're there for them and that they're not alone.

24. How do I find a support group for people with Psoriasis?

Finding a support group for people with psoriasis can be a helpful way to connect with others who understand the challenges of living with the condition. Here are some practical steps you can take to find a psoriasis support group in your area:

Ask your healthcare provider: Your dermatologist or primary care physician may be aware of local support groups for people with psoriasis. They may be able to provide you with contact information or even refer you to a specific group.

Search online: Many support groups have an online presence. You can search for psoriasis support groups on social media platforms such as Facebook or Meetup, or on websites like Psoriasis.org.

Contact national organizations: National organizations such as the National Psoriasis Foundation and the American Academy of Dermatology have local chapters that may offer support groups. Contacting these organizations can provide you with a list of support groups in your area.

Check with local hospitals: Some hospitals and medical centers have support groups for people with psoriasis. You can contact the hospital or medical center nearest you to see if they offer any support groups.

Consider online support groups: If you are not able to find a support group in your area or if you prefer to connect with others online, there are many online support groups for people with psoriasis. These groups can be accessed through social media platforms such as Facebook, or through websites like Psoriasis.org.

Once you have found a support group, you can attend meetings, share your experiences, and learn from others who understand what you are going through. It can also be a great way to find resources, advice and connect with others who may be experiencing similar issues.

Additionally, it's important to consider the format of the group, whether it's in-person, virtual or a combination of both and if there are any specific groups for certain sub-populations like children or specific ethnicities.

Definitely, finding a support group for people with psoriasis can be a valuable way to connect with others who understand the challenges of living with the condition and to learn more about managing your symptoms. By following these steps, you can find a support group that is right for you.

25. Can Psoriasis be passed through sexual intercourse?

There is no evidence to suggest that psoriasis can be transmitted through sexual intercourse. Psoriasis is not a contagious disease, and it cannot be spread through physical contact or through bodily fluids.

However, there are certain factors that can trigger a flare-up of psoriasis in some individuals. These include stress, infections, and certain medications. Sexual intercourse can cause stress in some people, and this stress can trigger a flare-up of psoriasis. Additionally, certain infections, such as strep throat, have been linked to psoriasis flare-ups.

It is also important to note that psoriasis can affect the genitals and can cause discomfort during sexual intercourse. In such cases, it is important to talk to a doctor about treatment options to manage the symptoms and improve sexual function.

Therefore, there is no evidence to suggest that psoriasis can be transmitted through sexual intercourse. However, stress and infections can trigger a flare-up of psoriasis. If you have psoriasis and experience discomfort during sexual intercourse, it is important to talk to a doctor about treatment options to manage the symptoms and improve sexual function.

SECTION 2

TREATMENT

26. Can Psoriasis be cured?

While there is currently no cure for psoriasis, there are many effective treatment options available that can help manage the symptoms and improve the quality of life for those living with the condition. However, it is important to note that psoriasis is a chronic condition that may require lifelong treatment. The treatment plan will be tailored to the individual, taking into account factors such as the severity of symptoms, the individual's overall health and medical history, and any other medical conditions that may be present.

27. How is Psoriasis treated?

One of the most popular natural treatment options for psoriasis is the use of topical creams and ointments that contain natural ingredients such as aloe vera, tea tree oil, and coconut oil. These ingredients have anti-inflammatory and moisturizing properties that can help to reduce redness, itching, and scaling associated with psoriasis. There is some evidence to support the use of these natural remedies in the treatment of psoriasis, but more research is needed to confirm their effectiveness.

Another natural treatment option for psoriasis is the use of dietary supplements, such as fish oil, vitamin D, and turmeric. Fish oil supplements contain omega-3 fatty acids, which have anti-inflammatory properties and can help to reduce the symptoms of psoriasis. Vitamin D supplements have also been shown to be beneficial in the treatment of psoriasis, as they can help to regulate the immune system and reduce the production of skin cells. Turmeric is another popular natural remedy for psoriasis, as it contains a compound called curcumin that has anti-inflammatory properties and can help to reduce redness and itching.

Medically, the most common treatment options for psoriasis include topical creams, ointments, and gels that contain corticosteroids, calcipotriene, or coal tar. These medications work by slowing down the production of skin cells and reducing inflammation. Topical corticosteroids are the most commonly used medication for psoriasis, as they are effective in reducing itching and redness, and can be used on a short-term basis. Calcipotriene is another commonly used medication that is similar to vitamin D, and can help to reduce the production of skin cells. Coal tar is also an effective treatment option for psoriasis, as it works by slowing down the production of skin cells and reducing itching and redness.

Another medical treatment option for psoriasis is the use of oral medications, such as methotrexate and acitretin. Methotrexate is a medication that is used to treat cancer and autoimmune diseases, and has been found to be effective in the treatment of psoriasis. Acitretin is a medication that is similar to vitamin A, and can help to reduce the production of skin cells and reduce inflammation.

In severe cases of psoriasis, light therapy or phototherapy may be recommended. This involves exposing the affected areas to UV light in a controlled setting. UVB light therapy is the most common type of phototherapy used to treat psoriasis, and it is effective in reducing itching and redness, and slowing down the production of skin cells.

In summary, psoriasis is a chronic skin condition that can be managed through a combination of natural and medical treatments. Natural remedies such as aloe vera, tea tree oil, and coconut oil may provide some relief from the symptoms of psoriasis, while medical treatment options such as topical creams, ointments, and gels, and oral medications, such as methotrexate and acitretin, can be more effective in managing the condition. Light therapy or phototherapy can also be used in severe cases of psoriasis. It is important to work closely with a healthcare provider to find the best treatment plan for an individual's specific needs and preferences.

28. How is Psoriasis diagnosed?

It is typically diagnosed by a medical professional through visual examination of the affected areas and a review of the patient's medical history. However, some individuals may also seek a natural diagnosis or treatment for their psoriasis.

Medical diagnosis of psoriasis typically involves a physical examination by a dermatologist, during which they will examine the skin for typical psoriasis symptoms such as red, scaly patches and raised, thickened plaques. They may also take a skin scraping or biopsy to confirm the diagnosis and rule out other potential skin conditions. Additionally, a medical professional may also review the patient's medical history, including any family history of psoriasis, to aid in the diagnosis.

On the other hand, natural diagnosis of psoriasis may involve a holistic approach, focusing on identifying underlying causes and triggers for the condition. This may include a dietary evaluation, as certain foods have been shown to aggravate psoriasis symptoms in some individuals. Stress management techniques may also be recommended, as stress is known to exacerbate psoriasis symptoms. Additionally, some practitioners may also recommend herbal or homeopathic remedies, supplements, or other natural treatments to help reduce symptoms and improve overall health.

Medical treatment for psoriasis typically involves a combination of topical and systemic therapies. Topical treatments, such as creams and ointments, are applied directly to the affected skin and can help reduce inflammation and slow the growth of new skin cells.

Systemic treatments, such as oral or injectable medications, work to reduce inflammation throughout the body and may be used in cases of severe or widespread psoriasis.

On the other hand, natural treatment for psoriasis typically involves lifestyle changes, dietary modifications, and herbal or homeopathic remedies. For example, some individuals may find that eliminating certain foods from their diet, such as gluten or nightshades, can improve their symptoms. Additionally, stress management techniques, such as yoga or meditation, may be recommended to reduce stress levels and improve overall well-being. Herbal remedies, such as aloe vera or turmeric, may also be recommended to help reduce inflammation and improve skin health.

Summarily, psoriasis is a chronic skin condition that can be diagnosed both naturally and medically. Medical diagnosis typically involves a physical examination and skin scraping or biopsy, while natural diagnosis may involve identifying underlying causes and triggers through dietary and lifestyle changes. Medical treatment typically involves topical and systemic therapies, while natural treatment typically includes lifestyle changes, dietary modifications, and herbal or homeopathic remedies. However, it is important to note that natural treatments may not be as effective as medical treatments and should be used in conjunction with medical treatments for best results. Additionally, it is important to consult with a medical professional before starting any natural treatments to ensure they are safe and appropriate for your individual case.

29. What are the side effects of Psoriasis treatment?

Topical treatments, such as corticosteroids, calcipotriene, and tazarotene, are commonly used to treat mild to moderate psoriasis. These medications work by reducing inflammation and slowing down the growth of skin cells. However, they can cause side effects such as skin irritation, burning, itching, and redness. Long-term use of topical corticosteroids can also lead to thinning of the skin, known as atrophy.

Light therapy, also known as phototherapy, involves exposing the affected skin to ultraviolet (UV) light. This treatment can be effective in reducing plaque size and improving symptoms, but it can also cause skin irritation, burning, and redness. In addition, long-term exposure to UV light can increase the risk of skin cancer.

Oral and injectable medications, such as methotrexate, acitretin, and biologic drugs, are used to treat moderate to severe psoriasis. These medications work by suppressing the immune system and slowing down the growth of skin cells. However, they can also cause side effects such as nausea, vomiting, diarrhoea, and liver damage. Biologic drugs, which are made from living cells, can also increase the risk of infections.

In addition to these side effects, psoriasis treatment can also have a psychological impact. The visible nature of psoriasis can lead to feelings of self-consciousness, embarrassment, and depression. Treatment options that involve exposing the skin to UV light can also make it difficult for patients to continue their normal daily activities.

Despite these side effects, psoriasis treatment is generally considered to be safe and effective. The benefits of treatment outweigh the risks, and most side effects can be managed with proper care and monitoring. Patients should work closely with their healthcare provider to find the right treatment plan that meets their individual needs and goals.

In conclusion, psoriasis treatment can cause a variety of side effects, including skin irritation, burning, itching, and redness, as well as more serious complications such as liver damage and skin cancer. However, with proper care and monitoring, the benefits of treatment outweigh the risks, and most side effects can be managed. Patients should work closely with their healthcare provider to find the right treatment plan that meets their individual needs and goals.

30. Can Psoriasis be prevented?

One of the most effective ways to prevent psoriasis flare-ups is to maintain a healthy lifestyle. This includes eating a balanced diet, getting regular exercise, and avoiding smoking and excessive alcohol consumption. These lifestyle changes can help to reduce inflammation in the body, which is a major contributing factor to psoriasis.

Another strategy that can help to prevent psoriasis flare-ups is to use a gentle skincare routine. This includes using non-irritating cleansers, moisturizers, and other skincare products that are specifically formulated for sensitive skin. Avoiding harsh soaps, scrubs, and other abrasive products can also help to reduce the risk of flare-ups.

Stress management is also important for preventing psoriasis flare-ups. Stress can trigger the release of inflammatory chemicals in the body, which can worsen psoriasis symptoms. Practicing relaxation techniques such as yoga, meditation, or deep breathing can help to reduce stress and prevent flare-ups.

There is also evidence that certain medications can be effective in preventing psoriasis flare-ups. For example, some studies have shown that topical retinoids can help to reduce the risk of psoriasis flare-ups. Additionally, some studies have found that methotrexate and cyclosporine, which are immunosuppressant medications, can be effective in preventing psoriasis flare-ups.

It is worthy of note to work closely with a dermatologist to develop an individualized treatment plan for managing psoriasis. This may include a combination of lifestyle changes, skincare strategies, stress management techniques, and medications. Regular follow-up appointments with a dermatologist can help to monitor symptoms, adjust treatment as needed, and prevent flare-ups.

While psoriasis cannot be prevented, there are several strategies that can be used to manage symptoms and reduce the risk of flare-ups. These include maintaining a healthy lifestyle, using a gentle skincare routine, managing stress, and working closely with a dermatologist to develop an individualized treatment plan. By following these strategies, individuals with psoriasis can better manage their condition and improve their overall quality of life.

31. How does diet affect Psoriasis?

Diet has been shown to play a role in the development and management of psoriasis. Studies have found that certain foods and nutrients may trigger or worsen symptoms, while others may have a beneficial effect.

One study found that a diet high in fruits, vegetables, and fish was associated with a lower risk of psoriasis, while a diet high in red and processed meats, refined grains, and sugar was associated with a higher risk. Another study found that a Mediterranean diet, which is rich in fruits, vegetables, whole grains, fish, and healthy fats, may improve psoriasis symptoms.

Some specific foods and nutrients that have been found to have a positive effect on psoriasis include:

Omega-3 fatty acids: These healthy fats, found in fish such as salmon and mackerel, have anti-inflammatory properties and may help reduce symptoms of psoriasis.

Vitamin D: This nutrient is important for skin health, and a deficiency has been linked to psoriasis. Foods that are high in vitamin D include fatty fish, mushrooms, and egg yolks.

Probiotics: These beneficial bacteria found in fermented foods such as yogurt, kefir, and sauerkraut may help improve gut health and reduce inflammation, which may in turn help improve psoriasis symptoms.

On the other hand, some foods and nutrients that have been found to trigger or worsen psoriasis include:

Gluten: This protein found in wheat, barley, and rye has been found to trigger psoriasis symptoms in some people. A gluten-free diet may be beneficial for those with psoriasis and gluten sensitivity.

Nightshades: Some people with psoriasis may be sensitive to the solanine found in nightshade vegetables such as tomatoes, peppers, and eggplants.

Alcohol: Consuming large amounts of alcohol may trigger psoriasis symptoms, and can also interact with some psoriasis medications.

It's important to note that different people may have different triggers and sensitivities, so it's best to work with a healthcare professional to figure out which foods and nutrients may be affecting your psoriasis. In general, a healthy diet that is rich in fruits, vegetables, whole grains, fish, and healthy fats, and low in processed foods, sugar, and alcohol, may be beneficial for managing psoriasis symptoms.

It's also worth mentioning that weight loss, specifically in those who are overweight or obese, may also help to reduce symptoms and improve overall health.

In summary, while there's no specific diet that's been proven to cure psoriasis, certain foods and nutrients may help to improve symptoms. Eating a healthy and balanced diet, rich in fruits and vegetables, fish, and healthy fats, and avoiding processed foods, sugar, and alcohol, may be beneficial for managing psoriasis.

32. Can Psoriasis affect my joint?

While psoriasis primarily affects the skin, it can also affect other parts of the body, including the joints. This is known as psoriatic arthritis.

Psoriatic arthritis is a form of inflammatory arthritis that affects individuals with psoriasis. It is characterized by inflammation and damage to the joints, resulting in pain, stiffness, and limited range of motion. The symptoms of psoriatic arthritis usually appear after the onset of psoriasis, but in some cases, it may develop before the skin symptoms appear.

The exact cause of psoriatic arthritis is unknown, but it is believed to be a combination of genetic and environmental factors. Research has shown that certain genes, such as HLA-Cw6 and IL-12B, are associated with an increased risk of developing psoriatic arthritis. Additionally, environmental factors, such as infection and stress, may trigger the development of psoriatic arthritis in individuals with a genetic predisposition.

Psoriatic arthritis affects different joints in different ways. In some cases, it can cause inflammation and damage to the fingers and toes, leading to a condition called dactylitis. This results in swelling and pain in the fingers and toes, making it difficult to perform everyday tasks. In other cases, psoriatic arthritis can affect the larger joints, such as the hips and knees, leading to stiffness and pain.

The diagnosis of psoriatic arthritis is based on a combination of clinical examination and laboratory tests. A physical examination is performed to assess the affected joints for swelling, pain, and limited range of motion. Laboratory tests, such as blood tests and x-rays, are used to confirm the diagnosis and assess the severity of the disease.

Treatment for psoriatic arthritis includes a combination of medications and lifestyle changes. Medications, such as non-steroidal anti-inflammatory drugs (NSAIDs) and disease-modifying antirheumatic drugs (DMARDs), are used to reduce inflammation and prevent joint damage. Biologic medications, such as TNF inhibitors and IL-17 inhibitors, are also used to target specific inflammatory pathways in the body.

Lifestyle changes, such as exercise and weight management, are also important for managing psoriatic arthritis. Regular exercise can help to maintain joint function and reduce pain and stiffness. Weight management is also important, as being overweight or obese can put additional stress on the joints, leading to increased pain and inflammation.

In conclusion, psoriasis is a chronic skin condition that can also affect the joints, leading to psoriatic arthritis. This form of inflammatory arthritis is characterized by inflammation and damage to the joints, resulting in pain, stiffness, and limited range of motion. The exact cause of psoriatic arthritis is unknown, but it is believed to be a combination of genetic and environmental factors. Treatment for psoriatic arthritis includes a combination of medications and lifestyle changes, such as exercise and weight management, to reduce inflammation and prevent joint damage. With proper treatment and management, individuals with psoriatic arthritis can lead a normal, active life.

33. How do I manage my Psoriasis on a daily basis?

Managing psoriasis on a daily basis can be a challenging task, but with the right approach, it is possible to effectively control symptoms and improve quality of life. Here are some practical tips for managing psoriasis on a daily basis:

Follow a consistent skincare routine: Keeping the skin moisturized is one of the most important things you can do to manage psoriasis. Use a moisturizer that contains ingredients such as ceramides, glycerin, or urea to help retain moisture in the skin. Applying a thick layer of moisturizer immediately after bathing can help lock in hydration.

Use medicated creams or ointments: Topical medications such as corticosteroids, vitamin D analogues, and retinoids can help reduce inflammation and slow down the growth of skin cells. These medications should be applied as directed by your healthcare provider and should not be used for prolonged periods of time without consulting with your healthcare provider.

Limit exposure to triggers: Certain triggers such as stress, smoking, and alcohol consumption can worsen psoriasis symptoms. Limiting exposure to these triggers can help reduce flare-ups.

Take good care of your nails: Psoriasis can affect the nails, causing them to become thickened and discolored. Keeping the nails trimmed and clean can help prevent infection and improve the appearance of the nails.

Exercise regularly: Exercise has been shown to have a positive impact on psoriasis symptoms. Regular physical activity can help reduce stress and improve overall health.

Follow a healthy diet: Eating a healthy diet that is rich in fruits, vegetables, and lean protein can help reduce inflammation and improve overall health. Avoiding foods that can trigger psoriasis symptoms such as processed foods and refined carbohydrates can also help.

Consider phototherapy: Phototherapy involves exposing the skin to ultraviolet (UV) light under the supervision of a healthcare provider. UV light can help reduce inflammation and slow down the growth of skin cells.

Consider taking oral medications: Oral medications such as methotrexate, acitretin, and cyclosporine can help reduce inflammation and slow down the growth of skin cells. These medications should be used under the supervision of a healthcare provider and should not be used for prolonged periods of time without consulting with your healthcare provider.

It is important to note that managing psoriasis is an ongoing process and may require adjustments based on individual needs and symptoms. It is important to work closely with your healthcare provider to develop an individualized treatment plan that is right for you.

In conclusion, managing psoriasis on a daily basis can be challenging, but it is possible to effectively control symptoms and improve quality of life by following a consistent skincare routine, using medicated creams or ointments, limiting exposure to triggers, taking good care of your nails, exercising regularly, following a healthy diet, considering phototherapy, and oral medications under the supervision of a healthcare provider. Working closely with your healthcare provider to develop an individualized treatment plan that is right for you is essential.

34. Can I have surgery with Psoriasis?

Yes, you can have surgery with psoriasis. However, it is important to note that certain precautions and considerations should be taken into account before and during the surgery to minimize the risk of complications.

Before undergoing surgery, it is important to inform your surgeon and anaesthesiologist about your psoriasis. This will allow them to take appropriate precautions, such as using topical creams or ointments to reduce the risk of infection and to minimize the risk of complications during the surgery.

During the surgery, your surgeon will take extra care to protect the affected areas of your skin, as well as to use sterile instruments and equipment. Additionally, your surgeon may use a special technique, such as a subcutaneous layer technique, to minimize the risk of post-operative infections.

In terms of evidence, a study published in the Journal of the American Academy of Dermatology found that patients with psoriasis who underwent surgery had similar outcomes to those without psoriasis. Additionally, another study published in the Journal of the American Academy of Dermatology found that patients with psoriasis who underwent surgery had a low risk of complications and a high rate of satisfaction with their outcomes.

However, it is important to note that some surgeries, such as skin grafts or wound closures, may be more challenging in patients with psoriasis due to the thickened and scaly nature of the skin. In these cases, your surgeon may recommend alternative treatment options or may need to take extra precautions to minimize the risk of complications.

Overall, while it is possible to have surgery with psoriasis, it is important to work closely with your surgeon and anaesthesiologist to minimize the risk of complications and to ensure the best possible outcome. It is also important to keep the psoriasis under control before and after the surgery to avoid complications.

In conclusion, patients with psoriasis can undergo surgery, but it is important to inform the surgeon and anaesthesiologist about your condition and to take appropriate precautions to minimize the risk of complications. Additionally, it is important to keep your psoriasis under control before and after the surgery to ensure the best possible outcome. With proper care and management, patients with psoriasis can have successful surgeries with minimal risk of complications.

35. Can I use natural remedies for my Psoriasis?

Psoriasis symptoms can be managed with the help of a variety of natural remedies. However, it is essential to keep in mind that there is insufficient scientific evidence to support these treatments' efficacy.

Aloe vera gel is a common natural treatment for psoriasis. Aloe vera can soothe irritated skin because it has anti-inflammatory properties. Aloe vera cream reduced the severity of psoriasis symptoms, according to a study published in the Journal of Dermatological Treatment.

Fish oil is another natural treatment for psoriasis that may be beneficial. Omega-3 fatty acids, which have anti-inflammatory properties, are abundant in fish oil. According to a study that was published in the Journal of the American Academy of Dermatology, taking fish oil supplements may help alleviate the symptoms of psoriasis.

Another natural treatment for psoriasis that may be beneficial is tea tree oil. Tea tree oil may help soothe irritated skin due to its anti-inflammatory and antimicrobial properties. A cream containing tea tree oil was found to be effective in reducing the severity of psoriasis symptoms in a study that was published in the Journal of Dermatological Treatment.

Psoriasis is just one of many conditions that traditional medicine has used turmeric to treat for centuries. Curcumin, a substance found in turmeric, has anti-inflammatory properties. A cream containing curcumin was found to be effective at reducing the severity of psoriasis symptoms in a study that was published in the Journal of Dermatological Treatment.

It is essential to keep in mind that, while these natural remedies may be helpful in reducing the severity of psoriasis symptoms, they should not be used in place of conventional medical care. If you have psoriasis, it's critical to collaborate with a doctor on a treatment plan that works best for you. Additionally, natural remedies should be used with caution because some may cause adverse effects or interact with other medications. Before beginning any new treatment, it is always recommended to speak with a medical professional.

In conclusion, natural remedies such as turmeric, fish oil, tea tree oil, and aloe vera gel may be helpful in managing psoriasis symptoms; however, more research is required to confirm their efficacy. Before starting any new treatment, it's important to talk to a doctor, and natural remedies should never be used in place of conventional medicine.

36. Can I use over-the-counter products for my Psoriasis?

Psoriasis can be treated with over-the-counter (OTC) medications. However, it is essential to keep in mind that the severity of your condition and the particular product you are using can have an impact on how effective these products are.

Moisturizers, salicylic acid, coal tar, and capsaicin are examples of over-the-counter products that may be beneficial for psoriasis. Moisturizers like lotions and creams can reduce scaling and soothe dry, irritated skin. Coal tar can help alleviate itching and inflammation, and salicylic acid is a keratolytic that can soften and remove scales. The chemical capsaicin, which comes from chili peppers, can also help reduce inflammation and itching.

It is essential to keep in mind that over-the-counter remedies for psoriasis should not be used in place of prescription medications. They work best when used in conjunction with a treatment plan that has been approved by a doctor. Before beginning any new treatment for psoriasis, including over-the-counter products, you should talk to your doctor.

Also, it's important to follow the directions for OTC products and don't use them on broken or irritated skin. You should stop using it and talk to your doctor if you have any side effects or don't see any improvement within a few weeks.

For mild to moderate cases of psoriasis, over-the-counter products may be helpful, but they may not be effective for severe cases. Topical corticosteroids, topical immunomodulators, and systemic medications may be required in these circumstances.

Over-the-counter products can be a useful complement to treatment for psoriasis; however, it's important to follow the directions and consult your doctor before using them.

It's also important to keep in mind that they may not be as effective as prescription medications in severe cases.

Before starting any new treatment for psoriasis, including over-the-counter (OTC) products, it's important to talk to a doctor. Although these products may be beneficial for mild to moderate psoriasis, they should not be used in place of prescription medications and may not be effective for severe cases.

Moisturizers, salicylic acid, coal tar, and capsaicin are examples of over-the-counter products that may be beneficial for psoriasis. Moisturizers like lotions and creams can reduce scaling and soothe dry, irritated skin. Coal tar can help alleviate itching and inflammation, and salicylic acid is a keratolytic that can soften and remove scales. The chemical capsaicin, which comes from chili peppers, can also help reduce inflammation and itching.

OTC products should only be used as directed, and they should not be applied to broken or irritated skin. You should stop using it and talk to your doctor if you have any side effects or don't see any improvement within a few weeks.

In a study that was published in the Journal of Dermatological Treatment, researchers discovered that a combination of salicylic acid and coal tar helped 60% of patients with psoriasis feel better. A moisturizer containing salicylic acid and urea was found to reduce itching and scaling in psoriasis patients in another study that was published in the Journal of the American Academy of Dermatology.

37. Can I use essential oils for my Psoriasis?

Essential oils have been used for centuries for their therapeutic properties and are known to have anti-inflammatory, anti-bacterial, and anti-fungal properties. They can also be used to reduce stress and promote relaxation, which can be beneficial for individuals with psoriasis.

There is some evidence that suggests that certain essential oils may be beneficial for individuals with psoriasis. For example, a study published in the Journal of Dermatology found that a blend of tea tree oil, neroli oil, and bergamot oil was effective in reducing the symptoms of psoriasis. Another study published in the Journal of the American Academy of Dermatology found that a cream containing a blend of essential oils, including tea tree oil, was effective in reducing the symptoms of psoriasis.

Tea tree oil is known for its anti-inflammatory and anti-bacterial properties, which make it a popular choice for treating skin conditions. It has been shown to be effective in reducing the redness and scaling associated with psoriasis.

Neroli oil is also known for its anti-inflammatory properties and has been shown to be effective in reducing the symptoms of psoriasis. In addition, neroli oil is known for its calming properties, which can be beneficial for individuals with psoriasis who experience stress and anxiety.

Bergamot oil is also known for its anti-inflammatory properties and has been shown to be effective in reducing the symptoms of psoriasis. It is also known for its uplifting properties, which can be beneficial for individuals with psoriasis who experience depression and anxiety.

It is important to note that essential oils should be used with caution and under the guidance of a healthcare professional. Essential oils should be diluted with a carrier oil, such as coconut oil, before being applied to the skin. They should not be used undiluted or ingested. It is also important to avoid using essential oils on broken or irritated skin, as they can cause skin irritation or allergic reactions.

Summarily, there is some evidence that suggests that certain essential oils may be beneficial for individuals with psoriasis. Essential oils, including tea tree oil, neroli oil, and bergamot oil, have been shown to be effective in reducing the symptoms of psoriasis. However, it is important to use essential oils with caution and under the guidance of a healthcare professional. It is also important to avoid using essential oils on broken or irritated skin, as they can cause skin irritation or allergic reactions. It's also important to remember that essential oils should be used in conjunction with other treatment options, such as topical creams and medications, as recommended by a healthcare professional.

38. Can I use tanning beds with Psoriasis?

UV light therapy, also known as phototherapy, is a common treatment for psoriasis. It involves exposing the skin to controlled amounts of UV light to slow down the growth of skin cells and reduce inflammation. UV light therapy can be administered in a number of ways, including natural sunlight, artificial UV light sources, and tanning beds.

Tanning beds are a type of artificial UV light source that emit UV rays similar to those found in natural sunlight. They are often used for tanning, but they can also be used for UV light therapy for psoriasis. However, it is important to note that tanning beds can be risky, as they emit UVA and UVB rays, both of which can cause skin cancer.

While tanning beds can be used for UV light therapy, they should be used with caution. The American Academy of Dermatology recommends that people with psoriasis avoid tanning beds and instead use UV light therapy administered by a dermatologist. This is because tanning beds emit UVA and UVB rays, both of which can cause skin cancer. Additionally, tanning beds do not emit UV light in a controlled manner, which can lead to overexposure and skin damage.

If you do decide to use a tanning bed for UV light therapy, it is important to do so under the guidance of a dermatologist. Your dermatologist can help you determine the appropriate dosage and frequency of UV light therapy, as well as monitor your skin for any changes or complications. It is also important to use a sunscreen with a minimum SPF of 30 on any exposed skin to protect against sunburn and skin cancer.

So, while tanning beds can be used for UV light therapy for psoriasis, it is important to do so with caution. Tanning beds emit UVA and UVB rays, both of which can cause skin cancer. Additionally, tanning beds do not emit UV light in a controlled manner, which can lead to overexposure and skin damage. If you do decide to use a tanning bed for UV light therapy, it is important to do so under the guidance of a dermatologist and to use a sunscreen with a minimum SPF of 30 on any exposed skin.

39. Can I use saunas with Psoriasis?

Saunas can be used by individuals with psoriasis, but it is important to be cautious and consult with a healthcare professional before using one.

Saunas have been shown to have anti-inflammatory properties, which can help to reduce the symptoms of psoriasis.

One study found that regular sauna sessions resulted in a significant reduction in the severity of psoriasis symptoms. The study participants were asked to take a sauna for 15 minutes, three times a week, for three months. At the end of the study, the participants reported a significant improvement in their skin condition.

Another study found that sauna therapy can be an effective treatment for psoriasis. The study participants were asked to take a sauna for 30 minutes, three times a week, for eight weeks. At the end of the study, the participants reported a significant improvement in their skin condition.

However, it is important to note that saunas can be dehydrating and can cause the skin to dry out. This can worsen psoriasis symptoms, so it is important to stay hydrated and use moisturizers before and after sauna sessions. Additionally, it is important to be cautious with the heat and humidity levels in the sauna, as high temperatures and humidity can irritate the skin.

It is also important to note that saunas should not be used as a replacement for traditional psoriasis treatments. Saunas should be used in conjunction with other treatments, such as topical creams or light therapy.

In conclusion, saunas can be used by individuals with psoriasis, but it is important to be cautious and consult with a healthcare professional before using one. Saunas have been shown to have anti-inflammatory properties, which can help to reduce the symptoms of psoriasis, but it is important to stay hydrated and use moisturizers before and after sauna sessions. Additionally, saunas should not be used as a replacement for traditional psoriasis treatments and should be used in conjunction with other treatments.

40. Can I use hot tubs with Psoriasis?

Hot tubs can be used by individuals with psoriasis, but it is important to understand the potential risks and benefits before use.

Hot tubs can provide relief for individuals with psoriasis as they can help to soothe the itching and inflammation associated with the condition. The warm water in the hot tub can help to increase blood flow to the skin, which can help to reduce inflammation and promote healing. Additionally, the heat in the hot tub can help to relax the muscles and promote a sense of relaxation and well-being.

However, it is important to note that hot tubs can also aggravate psoriasis symptoms if not used properly. The heat and humidity in the hot tub can dry out the skin, which can exacerbate symptoms of dryness and itching. Additionally, the chemicals used to clean and maintain the hot tub can irritate the skin and cause further inflammation.

To use a hot tub safely with psoriasis, it is important to take the following precautions:

- Keep the water temperature below 104 degrees Fahrenheit to avoid overheating the skin.

- Avoid prolonged exposure to the heat and humidity in the hot tub. A 10-15 minute soak is generally recommended.

- Avoid using harsh chemicals or soaps when cleaning the hot tub. Instead, use a mild, fragrance-free soap.

- Apply a moisturizer to the skin before and after using the hot tub to help keep the skin hydrated.

- Avoid using the hot tub if the skin is broken or inflamed.

It is also recommended to consult with a dermatologist before using hot tubs with psoriasis. They can provide personalized recommendations based on your specific condition and can help you to understand the potential risks and benefits of using a hot tub with psoriasis.

Really, hot tubs can be used by individuals with psoriasis, but it is important to understand the potential risks and benefits before use. By taking the appropriate precautions and consulting with a dermatologist, individuals with psoriasis can safely use hot tubs to help soothe their symptoms and promote healing.

41. How do I deal with the psychological effects of Psoriasis?

The physical symptoms of psoriasis, such as red, flaky patches of skin and itching, can be distressing, and the condition can also be associated with social stigmatization, leading to feelings of shame, isolation, and anxiety. However, there are a number of ways to manage the psychological effects of psoriasis, and evidence-based strategies can help individuals cope with the condition and improve their quality of life.

One effective way to manage the psychological effects of psoriasis is through cognitive-behavioral therapy (CBT). This type of therapy is designed to help individuals change negative thoughts and behaviors that can contribute to feelings of distress. For example, CBT can help individuals with psoriasis who feel self-conscious about their skin condition to develop strategies for managing negative thoughts and feelings, such as reframing negative self-talk and practicing mindfulness. A systematic review of randomized controlled trials found that CBT can improve mental health outcomes in individuals with psoriasis, including reducing depression and anxiety symptoms.

Another effective strategy for managing the psychological effects of psoriasis is through social support. Social support can help individuals with psoriasis to feel less alone and more connected to others, which can help to reduce feelings of isolation and anxiety. Support groups, both in-person and online, can provide a space for individuals with psoriasis to share their experiences and learn from others who are going through similar challenges. A systematic review of randomized controlled trials found that support groups can improve mental health outcomes in individuals with psoriasis, including reducing depression and anxiety symptoms.

Exercise is also a helpful strategy for managing the psychological effects of psoriasis. Regular physical activity can help to reduce stress, improve mood, and boost self-esteem. A systematic review of randomized controlled trials found that exercise can improve mental health outcomes in individuals with psoriasis, including reducing depression and anxiety symptoms. However, it is important to note that individuals with psoriasis should be mindful of the type of exercise they engage in, as activities that put excessive stress on the skin, such as heavy weightlifting or intense cardio, can aggravate psoriasis symptoms.

Lastly, medication and self-care treatment can help individuals to cope with psoriasis. Topical creams and ointments, as well as light therapy, can help to reduce the physical symptoms of psoriasis, which can in turn help to reduce feelings of distress. A systematic review of randomized controlled trials found that topical creams and ointments can improve mental health outcomes in individuals with psoriasis, including reducing depression and anxiety symptoms.

The psychological effects of psoriasis can be significant, but there are a number of evidence-based strategies that can help individuals to cope with the condition and improve their quality of life. These include cognitive-behavioral therapy, social support, exercise, and medication and self-care treatment. By utilizing these strategies and working with a healthcare professional, individuals with psoriasis can take steps to manage their symptoms and improve their overall well-being.

42. How do I deal with the social effects of Psoriasis?

Psoriasis's social effects can be difficult to manage, but there are ways to deal with them. In order to assist you in navigating the psoriasis's social effects, here are some concrete responses and justifications supported by evidence.

Share your knowledge of psoriasis with others: Knowing what psoriasis is and how to describe it can help you explain it to others and educate them about it. This may assist in reducing the condition's stigma and misperceptions. Psoriasis sufferers can be better understood and accepted through education and awareness campaigns.

Be honest and open with one another: Being honest and open about your condition with others can help alleviate feelings of isolation and shame. Additionally, it enables others to comprehend and support your requirements. Psoriasis sufferers' mental health can benefit from social support.

Find a group that can help: A sense of community and belonging can be gained by joining a support group. It can also provide a secure environment in which you can share your experiences and gain knowledge from those who have gone through similar ones. People who suffer from psoriasis have been shown in studies to benefit emotionally and in terms of quality of life from attending support groups.

Learn how to control stress: Psoriasis flares can be triggered by stress, so it's important to find ways to control it. This could be anything from yoga to meditation to exercise. Psoriasis sufferers can benefit from stress management strategies.

Make time for yourself: You can improve your mental and physical well-being by taking care of yourself. Healthy eating, getting enough sleep, and maintaining good hygiene are all examples of this. Self-care practices have been shown to improve psoriasis sufferers' symptoms and quality of life.

Get professional assistance: It may be beneficial to seek professional assistance if you are experiencing difficulties with psoriasis's social effects. Seeing a counselor, therapist, or psychologist is one option for this. Psychological interventions have been shown to improve psoriasis sufferers' emotional well-being and quality of life .

In conclusion, despite the fact that coping with the social effects of psoriasis can be difficult, there are strategies for managing and overcoming them. Finding a support group, learning to manage stress, practicing self-care, and seeking professional help are all effective strategies for managing the social effects of psoriasis. You can also educate yourself and others about psoriasis.

43. How do I cope with a flare-up of my Psoriasis?

Flare-ups, or exacerbations of symptoms, can be triggered by a variety of factors such as stress, infection, and changes in weather. Coping with a flare-up of psoriasis can be challenging, but there are several strategies that can help manage symptoms and reduce the impact on daily life.

One of the most effective ways to cope with a psoriasis flare-up is to maintain a consistent skincare routine. This includes using gentle, non-irritating soaps and moisturizers, avoiding harsh scrubs or exfoliants, and applying topical medications as prescribed by a healthcare provider. The National Psoriasis Foundation recommends using a moisturizer within three minutes of bathing or showering to lock in moisture and reduce itching. Additionally, using a humidifier in the home can also help keep skin hydrated and improve symptoms.

Another important strategy for coping with a psoriasis flare-up is to manage stress. Stress can worsen symptoms and trigger flare-ups, so it is important to find healthy ways to manage stress such as through exercise, meditation, or therapy. According to a study published in the Journal of the American Academy of Dermatology, regular exercise can improve symptoms of psoriasis and reduce the risk of flare-ups. Additionally, a study in the Journal of the European Academy of Dermatology and Venereology found that mindfulness-based stress reduction interventions can also improve symptoms of psoriasis.

Another way to cope with a psoriasis flare-up is to avoid triggers that can worsen symptoms. These triggers can include smoking, alcohol consumption, certain medications, and exposure to certain chemicals or irritants. According to a study in the Journal of the American Academy of Dermatology, smoking is a significant risk factor for psoriasis and can worsen symptoms. Additionally, alcohol consumption can also exacerbate symptoms and increase the risk of flare-ups.

Identifying and avoiding these triggers can help reduce the frequency and severity of flare-ups.

Lastly, it is important to work with a healthcare provider to develop an individualized treatment plan for psoriasis. This may include topical medications, phototherapy, or oral medications. A study in the Journal of the American Academy of Dermatology found that a combination of topical medications and phototherapy can be effective in managing psoriasis symptoms and reducing the risk of flare-ups. Additionally, oral medications such as methotrexate and biologic therapies can also be effective in managing symptoms and reducing the impact of flare-ups on daily life.

Therefore, coping with a flare-up of psoriasis can be challenging, but there are several strategies that can help manage symptoms and reduce the impact on daily life.

These strategies include maintaining a consistent skincare routine, managing stress, avoiding triggers, and working with a healthcare provider to develop an individualized treatment plan. By implementing these strategies, individuals with psoriasis can improve their symptoms and better manage the condition.

44. How do I address the physical pain caused by Psoriasis?

One of the most effective ways to address the physical pain caused by psoriasis is through the use of topical medications. Topical medications, such as creams and ointments, can be applied directly to the affected areas of the skin. These medications work by reducing inflammation and slowing down the growth of skin cells, which can help to reduce the redness, scaling, and itching associated with psoriasis. Examples of topical medications that are commonly used to treat psoriasis include coal tar, salicylic acid, and corticosteroids.

Another effective way to address the physical pain caused by psoriasis is through the use of phototherapy. Phototherapy involves exposing the affected areas of the skin to ultraviolet (UV) light. UV light can help to reduce inflammation and slow down the growth of skin cells, which can help to reduce the redness, scaling, and itching associated with psoriasis. Phototherapy can be administered in a dermatologist's office or at home using a UV lamp.

In addition to these treatments, lifestyle changes can also help to reduce the physical pain caused by psoriasis. For example, maintaining a healthy diet and exercise routine can help to improve overall health and reduce inflammation in the body. Stress management techniques, such as meditation and yoga, can also help to reduce the physical pain caused by psoriasis.

It is also important to note that people with psoriasis should avoid triggers that may worsen symptoms, such as alcohol, smoking, and certain medications.

Furthermore, there are also systemic medications that can be used to treat severe cases of psoriasis. These medications work by suppressing the immune system, which can help to reduce inflammation and slow down the growth of skin cells. Examples of systemic medications that are commonly used to treat psoriasis include methotrexate, cyclosporine, and biologics.

In summary, the physical pain caused by psoriasis can be addressed through the use of topical medications, phototherapy, lifestyle changes, and systemic medications. It is important to work with a dermatologist to find the most effective treatment plan for an individual's specific needs. It is also important to make lifestyle changes, avoid triggers, and maintain a healthy diet and exercise routine to improve overall health and reduce inflammation in the body.

45. How do I find a dermatologist experienced in treating Psoriasis?

Finding a dermatologist experienced in treating psoriasis can be a challenging task, but it is important to take the time to find the right doctor for your condition. There are several ways to go about finding a qualified dermatologist, and the following are some practical tips and reasons with evidence to help you find the right one for you.

Check the American Academy of Dermatology (AAD) website. The AAD is the largest professional organization for dermatologists in the United States, and they have a database of dermatologists on their website that you can search by location and specialty. This is a great resource for finding qualified dermatologists in your area who have experience treating psoriasis.

Ask for recommendations from your primary care physician. Your primary care physician may have recommendations for dermatologists in your area who have experience treating psoriasis. They may also have information about any specialists in your area who have a particular interest or expertise in treating psoriasis.

Ask for recommendations from others with psoriasis. There are many online communities for people with psoriasis, and these can be a great resource for finding a qualified dermatologist. Reach out to people in these communities and ask for recommendations for dermatologists who have helped them manage their psoriasis.

Research the dermatologist's qualifications and experience. Once you have a list of potential dermatologists, it is important to research their qualifications and experience. Look for a board-certified dermatologist who has experience treating psoriasis and has published research or articles on the topic. You can also check the dermatologist's website or social media profiles to see if they have any information about their experience treating psoriasis.

Schedule a consultation. Once you have narrowed down your list of potential dermatologists, schedule a consultation with each one. This will give you the opportunity to ask questions, discuss your concerns, and get a sense of the dermatologist's approach to treating psoriasis.

It is important to note that a study published in the Journal of the American Academy of Dermatology found that patients with psoriasis who saw a dermatologist had better outcomes and were more satisfied with their treatment than those who saw a primary care physician. This is because dermatologists have specialized training and experience in treating skin conditions like psoriasis, and are more likely to have access to the latest treatments and therapies.

In conclusion, finding a dermatologist experienced in treating psoriasis is crucial for managing the condition effectively. You can start by searching the American Academy of Dermatology website, ask for recommendations from your primary care physician, reach out to others with psoriasis, research the dermatologist's qualifications and experience, and schedule a consultation. With these tips and reasons, you are more likely to find a dermatologist who can help you manage your psoriasis and improve your quality of life.

46. How do I find financial assistance for Psoriasis treatment?

There are several ways to find financial assistance for psoriasis treatment, including the following:

Insurance coverage: Many insurance plans cover the cost of psoriasis treatment, including prescription medications, doctor visits, and procedures such as light therapy. Check with your insurance provider to see what is covered under your plan.

Patient assistance programs: Many pharmaceutical companies offer patient assistance programs for individuals who are unable to afford the cost of their medications. These programs may provide the medication for free or at a reduced cost.

Government programs: The government also offers financial assistance for those in need. Medicaid, for example, is a joint federal and state program that helps with medical costs for some people with limited income and resources.

Non-profit organizations: There are also non-profit organizations that provide financial assistance for medical treatments and medications. The National Psoriasis Foundation, for example, offers financial assistance to those in need.

Crowdfunding: There are also websites like GoFundMe, where people can raise money for medical treatments and procedures.

Negotiating with healthcare providers: Some healthcare providers may be willing to negotiate the cost of treatment, especially if you are paying out of pocket.

It is important to note that the financial assistance options available to you will depend on your individual circumstances and where you live. It is always good to check with your insurance provider, government programs and non-profit organizations to see what options are available to you.

Additionally, it is also important to talk to your healthcare provider about your treatment options. They may be able to recommend treatments that are more affordable or covered by insurance.

In conclusion, there are multiple options for financial assistance for psoriasis treatment, including insurance coverage, patient assistance programs, government programs, non-profit organizations, crowdfunding, and negotiating with healthcare providers. It is important to research the options available to you and speak with your healthcare provider and insurance provider to determine the best course of action.

47. How do I access clinical trials for Psoriasis?

Accessing clinical trials for psoriasis can be a challenging process, but it is an important step for those looking to find new treatments and therapies for this chronic skin condition. Clinical trials are research studies that test new medications, devices, and treatments in people to determine their safety and effectiveness. They are an important way to advance medical knowledge and improve patient outcomes.

The first step in accessing clinical trials for psoriasis is to find out if there are any current trials that are recruiting participants. This information can be found through a variety of sources, including:

ClinicalTrials.gov: This is a website maintained by the National Institutes of Health (NIH) that lists all clinical trials that are currently recruiting participants in the United States. You can search for trials by condition, location, and other criteria.

Pharmaceutical company websites: Many pharmaceutical companies conduct clinical trials for psoriasis and other conditions. You can search their websites for information about current trials.

Psoriasis organizations: Many psoriasis organizations, such as the National Psoriasis Foundation, have information on current clinical trials.

Your healthcare provider: Your healthcare provider may also know of current clinical trials that are recruiting participants.

Once you have found a trial that you are interested in, you will need to determine if you are eligible to participate. Eligibility criteria vary from trial to trial, but typically include factors such as age, diagnosis, and current treatment. It is important to read the trial's inclusion and exclusion criteria carefully to ensure that you meet all the requirements.

After determining your eligibility, the next step is to contact the trial's study coordinator. They will be able to provide you with more information about the trial, including how to enroll. They will also be able to answer any questions you may have about the trial.

It is important to note that clinical trials are not right for everyone. They may require a significant time commitment, and some trials may require that participants stop taking other medications or treatments.

Additionally, clinical trials are often conducted at specific locations, so you may need to travel to participate.

It is also important to understand that there is a chance that the treatment being tested may not be effective, or that you may experience side effects. However, the benefits of participating in a clinical trial include the possibility of receiving new treatments that are not yet available to the general public, and the opportunity to contribute to the advancement of medical knowledge.

In conclusion, accessing clinical trials for psoriasis can be a challenging process, but it is an important step for those looking to find new treatments and therapies for this chronic skin condition. The first step is to find out if there are any current trials that are recruiting participants, and then determine if you are eligible to participate. It is important to understand that clinical trials are not right for everyone and may require a significant time commitment, but they can offer the possibility of receiving new treatments and the opportunity to contribute to the advancement of medical knowledge.

48. How do I stay up-to-date on the latest Psoriasis research?

Staying up-to-date on the latest psoriasis research is important for both patients and healthcare professionals as it allows for the most current and effective treatment options to be utilized. Here are some practical ways to stay informed:

Follow reputable organizations and journals: Organizations such as the National Psoriasis Foundation and the International Psoriasis Council regularly update their websites with the latest research and news in psoriasis. Additionally, journals such as the Journal of the American Academy of Dermatology and the Journal of Psoriasis and Psoriatic Arthritis regularly publish articles on psoriasis research.

Attend conferences and seminars: Conferences and seminars on psoriasis and related topics provide an opportunity to hear about the latest research and treatment options from experts in the field. These events also provide a platform for networking with other professionals and patients.

Sign up for newsletters and alerts: Many organizations and journals offer newsletters and alerts that notify subscribers of new research and articles related to psoriasis. This can be a convenient way to stay informed without having to actively search for new information.

Join online communities: Online communities such as forums and social media groups dedicated to psoriasis provide a platform for patients and healthcare professionals to discuss the latest research and treatment options. This can also provide a support system for those dealing with the condition.

Consult with a healthcare professional: Regularly consulting with a healthcare professional who specializes in psoriasis can provide patients with the most current and effective treatment options. Healthcare professionals also have access to resources and information that may not be readily available to the general public.

It is important to note that not all research on psoriasis is created equal. It is important to critically evaluate the quality and validity of the research before making any decisions based on it. This can be done by looking at the sample size, methods used, and funding sources of the research. Additionally, it is important to consult with a healthcare professional before making any changes to treatment plans based on new research.

In summary, staying up-to-date on the latest psoriasis research can be done through a variety of methods such as following reputable organizations and journals, attending conferences and seminars, signing up for newsletters and alerts, joining online communities, and consulting with a healthcare professional. It is important to critically evaluate the research and consult with a healthcare professional before making any changes to treatment plans. By staying informed, patients and healthcare professionals can utilize the most current and effective treatment options for psoriasis.

49. How do I advocate for more resources and support for people with Psoriasis?

Advocating for more resources and support for individuals with psoriasis can be done in a variety of ways, including educating oneself on the condition, building relationships with community leaders and healthcare professionals, and utilizing social media and other platforms to raise awareness.

Firstly, it is important to understand the impact that psoriasis can have on an individual's physical and mental well-being. According to a study published in the Journal of the American Academy of Dermatology, individuals with psoriasis have an increased risk of developing depression, anxiety, and suicidality. Additionally, psoriasis can have a significant impact on an individual's quality of life and can lead to decreased work productivity and increased healthcare costs.

One way to advocate for more resources and support is to educate oneself on the condition and its impact on individuals. This includes understanding the various treatment options available, as well as the barriers that individuals with psoriasis may face in accessing care. This knowledge can be used to inform discussions with healthcare professionals, policymakers, and community leaders.

Another way to advocate for more resources and support is to build relationships with community leaders and healthcare professionals. This can include reaching out to local politicians, healthcare providers, and advocacy organizations to share information about the impact of psoriasis and the need for increased resources and support. By building these relationships, individuals can work together to increase awareness of the condition and advocate for changes in policy and practice.

Social media can also be an effective tool for raising awareness and advocating for more resources and support for individuals with psoriasis. By sharing personal stories and information about the condition, individuals can help to educate others and raise awareness of the need for increased resources and support. Additionally, social media can be used to connect with other individuals with psoriasis and advocacy organizations, which can provide a sense of community and support.

In summary, advocating for more resources and support for individuals with psoriasis involves educating oneself on the condition, building relationships with community leaders and healthcare professionals, and utilizing social media and other platforms to raise awareness. By highlighting the impact of psoriasis on individuals' physical and mental well-being, as well as the barriers to accessing care, individuals can work to increase resources and support for those affected by psoriasis.

50. What is the best advice you can give someone diagnosed with Psoriasis?

If you have been diagnosed with psoriasis, it is important to understand that it is a chronic condition that cannot be cured, but can be managed effectively with proper treatment and self-care. It is also important to have a positive attitude and to not let psoriasis define who you are as a person.

One practical tip for managing psoriasis is to establish a regular skincare routine that includes gentle cleansing, moisturizing, and protecting your skin from the sun. Studies have shown that regular use of moisturizers can improve the appearance and severity of psoriasis symptoms. Additionally, using a sunscreen with a minimum SPF of 30 can help protect your skin from UV rays, which can worsen psoriasis.

Another important aspect of managing psoriasis is to maintain a healthy lifestyle, including eating a balanced diet, getting regular exercise, and avoiding smoking and excessive alcohol consumption. Studies have shown that maintaining a healthy weight, eating a diet rich in fruits, vegetables, and fish, and avoiding processed foods can improve psoriasis symptoms.

Another tip is to seek out emotional and psychological support. Psoriasis can have a significant impact on a person's emotional well-being, and it's important to have people around you who understand what you're going through and can offer support. You may also want to consider seeing a counselor or therapist who can help you cope with the emotional and psychological impact of psoriasis.

Lastly, it's important to stay informed about the latest psoriasis treatments and to work closely with your healthcare provider to find the best treatment plan for you. With the right treatment and self-care, you can manage your psoriasis and live a full and active life.

Good Job on the completion of this book!

Knowledge is Power!

Now that you are aware, you are out of the trap of fear!

You may want to read any of my other books

HEALTHY HABITS FOR MEN!

HEALTHY HABITS FOR WOMEN!

NOTIFICATION FATIGUE!

Check them out!

Dr. Chris Allan

www.ingramcontent.com/pod-product-compliance
Lightning Source LLC
Chambersburg PA
CBHW071221260726
48653CB00042B/1476